EAT TO OVERCOME ILLNESS:

What to eat to be healthy

By

Jim K. Call

TABLE OF CONTENT

INTRODUCTION

You may feel alive, process information, sleep, move, and unwind every day thanks to your body. Eating the right foods makes it easier for your body to maintain you. One of the "three cornerstones of health"—nutritious eating—bolsters your immune system.

A disease can be avoided with the help of a nutritious diet. A healthy diet can help you wade off bacterial and viral illnesses, improve your mood and energy levels, and lessen feelings of hopelessness and anxiety, but it can't replace social isolation or mask-wearing around other people. It might be a way of life rather than a strict diet or program based on calorie counting.

Consuming a healthy diet, even in tiny doses, increases your body's resistance to disease. See why your body responds differently to various meals when battling invaders by reading on.

Inflammation is under the control of the body's immune system. Even in the absence of external intruders, your immune system can still cause inflammation. This is an overreaction that could be dangerous.

Your body's defenses against foreign invaders, such as the coronavirus, are hampered by excessive inflammation. Try these meals to boost your immunity and reduce inflammation. Certain fruits and vegetables, such as onions, celery, berries, tomatoes, and apples, reduce inflammation. Even while there isn't a single meal, vitamin, or supplement that can stop infections, eating a balanced diet can help your body fight off disease. Everything boils down to equilibrium. Supplements containing vitamins and minerals might be helpful, but only if you aren't regularly getting enough of those nutrients.

Supplements may be hazardous if you take too many of them at once. The secret to everything is moderation. If you have any chronic or underlying medical conditions, speak with your primary care physician before beginning any new pharmaceutical regimen.

You will learn simple strategies for keeping up a healthy diet from this book. Simply take a seat back, relax, and benefit from this game-changing strategy.

CHAPTER 1

Who is able to eat well?

Eating healthily is defined as adhering to a balanced eating pattern that includes a series of nutrient-dense meals and drinks. It also means consuming the right amount of calories—not going over or under. You may uphold a healthy weight by eating a balanced, healthful diet. Your immune system may be weakened by certain essential minerals, including zinc, iron, selenium, and vitamins A, B, C, and E.

It offers defense against numerous chronic noncommunicable diseases, including cancer, diabetes, and heart disease. Eating a range of foods and limiting your intake of sugar, salt, saturated fat, and trans fats produced artificially are all part of a balanced diet. A varied range of foods make up a healthy diet. Here are a few instances:

Staples include starchy tubers, roots (potato, yam, taro, or cassava), and cereals (wheat, barley, rye, maize, or rice).

Legumes include beans and lentils.

Fruits and vegetables.

Foods that come from animals (meat, fish, eggs, and milk).

In addition to encouraging healthy growth, breastfeeding may offer long-term health benefits, such as a decreased risk of noncommunicable diseases and overweight/obesity in later life. From birth to six months of age, a newborn must only be fed breast milk as part of a balanced diet. It's also crucial to nurse your child until he or she is two years old or older and to start offering a variety of safe and nourishing supplemental meals at six months of age.

Eating the right amount of calories for your activity level is essential to a balanced diet because it balances the energy you store.

Eating healthily does not exist. Instead, it entails prioritizing your health by feeding your body meals high in nutrients. You ought to use as much energy as you produce. You will acquire weight if you eat more calories than your body needs since excess energy is stored as fat. If you consume too little food and liquids, you will lose weight.

In order to guarantee that your diet is well-balanced and that your body gets all the nutrients it needs, you should also eat a variety of meals. A man's daily calorie intake should be approximately 2,500 (10,500 kilojoules). Approximately 2,000 calories (8,400 kilojoules) should be consumed daily by women.

The accuracy is that maintaining a healthy diet need not be difficult. You may eat your favorite foods and fuel your body at the same time. Food should be savored, not feared, counted, weighed, and monitored, after all.

Why is it vital to eat healthily?

Above all, food is your source of energy and gives your body the calories and minerals it needs to function. If you don't get enough calories or certain nutrients in your diet, your health may suffer.

In a similar vein, overindulging in calories can lead to weight gain. A person who is obese have a significantly increased risk of contracting conditions, including type 2 diabetes, obstructive sleep apnea, and issues with their hearts, livers, and kidneys.

In addition, the caliber of your diet affects your longevity, mental health, and susceptibility to illness. Diets rich in whole, nutrient-dense foods have been associated with longer lifespans and disease prevention, whereas diets substantial in ultra-processed foods have been associated to increase mortality and a higher risk of diseases, including cancer and heart disease. Processed food-heavy diets may also increase the risk of depressive symptoms, particularly in individuals who engage in less activity.

Additionally, you're probably not receiving enough nutrients if your current diet is substantial in ultra-processed foods and drinks like soda, fast food, and sugary grains but low in real foods like vegetables, nuts, and fish. This can be deleterious to your overall health.

Healthy eating is important because it fuels your body, provides the nutrients it needs, lowers your risk of illness, increases longevity, and promotes optimal mental and physical well-being. Does eating healthily require adhering to a specific diet? Of course not!

Most people don't need to adhere to any particular diet in order to feel their best, even if other people need or prefer to avoid specific foods or diets for health-related reasons. That is not to say that there cannot be benefits to some dietary practices. While some people thrive on high-carb diets, others feel healthiest when they follow a low-carb diet.

Eating properly generally has nothing to do with adhering to strict diet plans or dietary specifications. "Healthy eating" simply refers to prioritizing your physical well-being by consuming nourishing foods for your body.

The specifics will change according to your area, budget, social and cultural norms, and personal preferences.

Essentials Of Nutrition: Micronutrient Ratio

Minerals and vitamins are the two categories into which micronutrients fall. Even though tiny amounts are all that are needed, they play a vital role in human growth and health by controlling vital processes like metabolism, heart rate, cellular pH, and bone density. In children, micronutrient deficiencies can lead to stunted growth, and in adults, they can increase the risk of numerous ailments. If people do not eat enough micronutrients, they might develop diseases, including rickets (a lack of vitamin D), scurvy (a lack of vitamin C), and osteoporosis (a lack of calcium).

They facilitate the body's production of hormones, enzymes, and other substances needed for healthy growth and development, among other functions. Deficiencies in iron, vitamin A, and iodine are the most common in the globe, particularly in children and expectant mothers. Micronutrient examples

Macronutrients can be found in common foods like fruits and vegetables, just as micronutrients.

Micronutrients include vitamins like the ones listed below:

• Vitamin B1. Thiamine, or vitamin B1, is a necessary component in the process that turns food into energy. Black beans, white rice, and morning cereals with added nutrients are a few food examples.

• Vitamin B2. This vitamin, also referred to as riboflavin, helps cells function, produce energy, and break down fat. Foods include things like milk, fat-free yogurt, and instant oats.

• Vitamin B3. Niacin, or vitamin B3, is a B vitamin that is frequently used to make energy from food. Foods include salmon, tuna, turkey breast, and chicken breast.

• Vitamin B5. Pantothenic acid, another name for this vitamin, helps the body produce fatty acids. Avocados, shiitake mushrooms, and sunflower seeds are a few culinary examples.

• Vitamin B6. Pyridoxine, another name for vitamin B6, helps produce red corpuscle and releases sugar from stored carbohydrates for energy. Foods include potatoes, tuna, and chickpeas.

• Vitamin B7. Also referred to as biotin, it aids in the metabolism of glucose, amino acids, and fatty acids. Among the culinary options are sweet potatoes, salmon, eggs, and pork chops.

• Vitamin B9. Likewise known as folate. Cell division cannot occur normally without vitamin B9. Foods include things like asparagus, white rice, fortified morning cereals, and spinach.

• Vitamin B12. Cobalamin, another name for vitamin B12, is an essential component of red blood cells and supports healthy brain and nervous system function. Foods include things like salmon, yogurt, milk, and beef liver.

• Vitamin C. Ascorbic acid, another name for vitamin C, is a necessary precursor to neurotransmitters and collagen. Foods include oranges, grapefruits, kiwis, and red peppers.

Some minerals that are good examples of micronutrients are:

• A mineral is calcium. This mineral supports healthy muscle function and the development of strong bones and teeth. Foods include things like milk, cheese, yogurt, and orange juice.

• A mineral is magnesium. This mineral aids in blood pressure regulation and can be found in foods such as spinach, almonds, and pumpkin seeds.

• A mineral is sodium. Salt is necessary to keep your blood pressure and fluid balance stable.

• A mineral is potassium. Potassium plays a role in nerve and muscle transmission. Foods including prunes, raisins, lentils, and apricots contain potassium.

Nutrient density

Calories are generally the first thing that springs to mind when you think of eating healthfully. Calorie intake is important, but your main priority should be nourishment.

This is due to the fact that in order to survive, your body requires nutrients, including protein, carbs, fat, vitamins, and minerals. While nutritional units are present in all foods, not all foods are nutrient-dense. "Nutrient density" is the ratio of a food's nutrients to its calories.

For instance, a box of mac and cheese or a candy bar may be high in calories but lacking in fiber, protein, vitamins, and minerals. Foods with the labels "low calorie" or "diet-friendly" may be high in nutrients yet low in calories. For example, compared to whole eggs, egg whites contain significantly less fat and calories. In contrast, a whole egg contains 5-21% of the Daily recommended intake for iron, phosphorus, zinc, choline, and vitamins A and B12. An egg white, on the other hand, comprises 1% or fewer of these nutrients. This is because eggs have a high-fat, healthful yolk.

Moreover, while a lot of fruits and vegetables and other nutrient-dense foods are low in calories, a lot of other foods, like almonds, full-fat yogurt, avocados, egg yolks, and fatty fish, are high in calories. That's totally okay! Foods that are high in calories may not necessarily mean they are bad for you. In a similar vein, a food item is not necessarily nutritious just because it has little calories.

The purpose of healthy eating is lost if you choose meals only based on their calorie content.

Eat meals high in nutrients, such as protein, fiber, healthy fats, vitamins, and minerals, as an overall rule of thumb. Veggies, fruits, nuts, seeds, beans, fish, and eggs are some of these foods.

Variety in diet

Another aspect of eating well is ingesting a variety of foods or dietary diversity. A varied diet includes a range of foods from several dietary groups, including grains, fruits and vegetables, dairy products, lipids, and lean proteins. This assortment ensures that you obtain an extensive array of nutrients, vitamins, minerals, and other essential elements that support overall well-being.

Eating a varied diet keeps your body weight in check, supports good gut flora, and guards against chronic disease.

However, it could be difficult to eat a variety of meals if you're a picky eater. If this is the case, gradually introduce different dishes. If you're not a big veggie eater, start small by incorporating your favorite veggie into one or two daily meals and work your way up.

Research indicates that the more times you are exposed to a food, the more likely you are to develop accustomed to it, even though you may not enjoy trying new foods.

Dietary diversity has the following benefits:

1. Nutrient intake: Eating a varied diet guarantees that you get a range of important vitamins and minerals because different foods contain different nutrients.

2. Taste and enjoyment: Varying up your meals can add delight to your diet and prevent you from growing bored with the same old foods.

3. Nutritional balance: You can maintain a balanced intake of micronutrients (vitamins and minerals) and macronutrients (carbs, proteins, and fats) by eating a varied diet.

4. Benefits to health: Eating a variety of meals has been associated with a decreased risk of chronic illnesses and nutritional deficiencies.

5. Gut Health: Eating a varied diet can help improve the bacteria in the gut, which is good for digestion and overall health.

Ratio of Macronutrients

The proportionate amounts of the three main macronutrients in your diet—carbs, proteins, and fats—are referred to as macronutrient ratios. This ratio could change depending on your dietary goals and needs.

1. Energy-producing carbohydrates: can make up a sizable portion of your daily caloric intake. Common sources include fruits, vegetables, grains, and legumes. Although recommendations for carbohydrate consumption vary, they typically range from 45% to 65% of total kilocalories consumed daily.

2. Proteins: A range of biological functions, including development and repair, depend on proteins. Lean meat, chicken, fish, lentils, and dairy products can all provide them. Although the recommended daily intake of protein varies, it usually ranges from 10% to 35% of total calories.

3. Fats: Dietary fats are essential for cell health, energy production, and the absorption of fat-soluble vitamins. Rich sources of fat include nuts, oils, avocados, and fatty fish. 20–35% of total calories per day should come from dietary fat.

The ideal ratio of macronutrients for you depends on factors including age, gender, degree of exercise, and food preferences.

The three main nutrients that are received through eating are protein, fat, and carbohydrates. (Fiber falls into the category of carbohydrates.

Generally speaking, divide your meals and snacks equally across the three. For example, adding fat and protein to foods high in fiber makes dishes seem more substantial and appealing. For instance, if you're having fruit as a snack, combining it with a tablespoon of nut butter or a little piece of cheese will keep you fuller for longer. Still, it's okay if you don't always have a balanced diet. Most people don't need to track their macros or adhere to a set diet of macronutrients, with the exception of athletes, those aiming for specific body composition, and those who must gain muscle or fat for certain medical conditions.

Moreover, obsessing about staying within a predetermined macro range and tracking macros can result in disordered eating and an unhealthy fixation with food and calories. It's important to remember that some people do well on diets that are high in fat and low in carbohydrates, or vice versa. However, macronutrient tracking is usually not necessary, even on these diets.

Eating low-carb meals like non-starchy vegetables, proteins, and fats more frequently than high-carb items will usually be sufficient if you feel your best on a low-carb diet, for example.

CHAPTER 2

The Threats of Eating Processed Foods

What Exactly Is Processed Food?

Any food that has been changed during preparation to make it more convenient, shelf-stable, or delicious is considered processed. Some foods are far more processed than others. Although a bagged salad or pre-cut green beans are technically processed, they are just a little processed because their natural form has not changed. In other words, it seems to be the same as it would in nature. A pack of macaroni and cheese or a microwaveable supper, on the other hand, is severely processed (also known as hyper-processed) since they have been chemically changed with artificial flavors, additives, and other components.

By the time they reach our plates, most meals have been prepared in some form. However, the concern about processed food is not about canned tomatoes or canned tuna, which are treated to preserve freshness and nutrition.

More intensively processed goods, such as crackers, canned spaghetti sauces, and cake mixes, are causing worry.

Cutting less on ultra-processed meals is one of the best strategies to enhance your diet. You don't have to fully shun processed meals. In certainty, many healthy foods, such as shelled almonds, canned beans, and frozen fruits and veggies, have been processed in a way.

In contrast, substantially processed foods and refreshments such as soda, baked goods, candy, sugary cereals, and many packaged snack foods contain few, if any, whole food components. Heavy fructose corn syrup, hydrogenated oils, and artificial sweeteners are common components in these products. They typically contain components that, if taken in excess, might be harmful, such as saturated fats, added sugar, and salt. These foods are also lower in fiber and nourishment content than whole foods.

Diets heavy in ultra-processed foods have been associated to an increased risk of depression, hypertension, obesity, and a variety of other issues.

Diets low in these items and heavy in full, nutrient-dense foods, conversely, have the opposite impact, guarding against illness, extending longevity, and improving general physical and mental well-being.

As a result, it is advisable to prioritize nutrient-dense diets, particularly vegetables and fruits.

Ultra-processed foods include the following:

• frozen or ready-to-eat meals

• baked products (such as pizza, cakes, and pastries)

• pre-packaged breads

• cheese items that have been treated

• cereals for breakfast

• crudites and chips

• sweets and ice cream

• ready-to-eat noodles and soups

• foods that have been reconstituted, such as sausages, nuggets, fish fingers, and processed ham

• sodas and other sugary beverages

The Health Dangers of Highly Processed Foods

Ultra-processed foods have several possible health consequences, including:

1. An increased chance of cancer.

2. Excess sugar, salt, and fat. Processed foods frequently include harmful quantities of added sugar, salt, and fat. These components improve the flavor of the food we consume, but too many of them cause major health problems such as obesity, heart disease, high blood pressure, and diabetes.

3. Nutritious value is lacking. Because heavy processing depletes many foods of their essential nutrients, many foods are now fortified with fiber, vitamins, and minerals.

4. High in calories and addictive. It is all too simple to overeat unhealthy foods and consume more calories than we realize. A cookie, for example, has roughly 50 calories, but a cup of green beans has just 44 calories.

These processed meals are also intended to activate our brain's "feel-good" dopamine area, causing us to seek more of them in the future.

5. It is easier to digest. Processed foods are simpler to digest than whole, unprocessed meals. That implies our bodies use less energy (hint: calories) to digest them. We expend half as many calories digesting processed foods as we do unprocessed foods. This, along with the high-calorie density of processed meals in general, can make it simple to gain weight.

6. Packed with artificial substances. Approximately 5,000 chemicals are added to our diet. The majority of them have never been tested by anyone other than the firm that employs them. This comprises color, texture, taste, and odor modifiers, as well as compounds like preservatives and sweeteners.

7. Carbohydrates that have been refined. Carbohydrates are an important part of every diet. Carbohydrates from whole foods, on the other hand, have significantly more health advantages than processed carbs.

The body quickly breaks down sophisticated or simple carbohydrates, making blood sugar and insulin levels to spurt. When these levels reduce, a person may suffer food cravings and debility.

Consuming sophisticated carbohydrates is connected with an increased risk of type 2 diabetes because they stimulate frequent spikes and drops in blood sugar.

Highly processed meals include a lot of refined carbs.

Carbohydrates that are good for you include:

complete grains

vegetables

fruits

legumes and pulses

8. Trans fat. Ultra-processed foods are frequently heavy in unhealthy, low-cost fats. For example, they frequently contain refined seed or vegetable oils, which are simple to use, affordable, and long-lasting.

Manufacturers produce synthetic trans fats by adding hydrogen to liquid vegetable oils, causing them to solidify.

Trans fats contribute to increased irritation in the body. They also increase low-density lipoprotein, or "worsen," cholesterol levels while decreasing compactness lipoprotein, or "good" cholesterol levels.

Trans fat consumption has been associated to a significant risk of heart disease, stroke, and type 2 diabetes. Avoiding processed meals is the greatest approach to prevent refined oils and trans fats. These can be substitute with healthier options such as coconut oil or olive oil.

Reducing Your Consumption of Processed Foods

Even if you wanted to, eliminating all severely processed items from your diet would be quite rigid. However, there are several things you may take to limit your consumption of processed foods:

1. Examine the label. The longer a food's ingredient list, the more processed it is. If the majority of the components are difficult-to-pronounce chemicals rather than genuine food, it's a fair bet that the meal has been severely processed.

2. Shop the food store's outside aisles. Most grocery store center aisles are crammed with processed packaged goods and ready-

made delicacies. Increase your purchases from the vegetable and dairy aisles.

2. Select meats that have been lightly processed. Choose less processed meats (e.g., shellfish, chicken breast) and avoid severely processed meats (e.g., sausage, cured meats like bacon).

3. Begin gently. It is OK to gradually replace processed foods in your diet with more fresh meals. It may increase your likelihood of sticking with these adjustments in the long run.

4. Prepare more meals at home. While traveling, you may not always be in charge of your nutrition, but you are at home. Cook a larger quantity of frozen meals and freeze the leftovers, or make your salad dressing.

While many elements of our health might be complex, consuming less processed food does not have to be one of them. When in doubt, begin with actual food.

Reduce your use of drinks, processed meats, sweets, ice cream, fried meals, fast food, and heavily processed, packaged snacks to boost your health and reduce your risk of some illnesses.

You do not, however, have to fully elude these items all of the time. Instead, strive to prioritize whole, nutrient-dense meals such as vegetables, fruits, nuts, seeds, grains, and seafood, reserving heavy processed foods and beverages for infrequent treats.

Ice cream and sugar can be part of a healthy, versatile diet, but they should not account for a huge portion of your calorie consumption. You should restrict your intake of ultra-processed foods and beverages such as candy, soda, and sugary cereals, but this does not imply you should eliminate them from your diet.

How to Make Eating Healthy Work for You

Food is one of many jigsaw pieces that make up your day-to-day existence. Between journeying, working, family or social obligations, errands, and many other everyday responsibilities, eating may be the last thing on your mind.

Making food a priority is the first step in eating a better diet. This does not imply that you must spend hours on meal preparation or cooking complicated meals, but it does entail some thinking and work, especially if you own a bustling itinerary.

Going to the grocery store once or twice a week, for example, will help ensure that you have healthy selections in your fridge and pantry. As a result, having a well-supplied kitchen makes it much easier to choose healthy meals and snacks.

Store up on the following items when you go food shopping:

- Fruits and vegetables, both fresh and frozen
- Reservoirs of protein such as chicken, eggs, fish, and tofu
- Carbohydrate sources such as canned beans and whole grains
- White potatoes, sweet potatoes, and nut squash are samples of starchy vegetables.
- Reservoirs of fat such as avocados, olive oil, and full-fat yogurt
- Pecans, grains, nut butter, hummus, olives, and dried fruit are all healthful and simple snack components.

When it comes to lunchtime, keep things simple and think in threes:

Protein: eggs, poultry, fish, or a plant-based alternative such as tofu

- Fat sources include olive oil, nuts, grains, nut butter, avocado, cheese, and full-fat yogurt.
- Fiber-rich carbohydrates include starchy alternatives such as sweet potatoes, oats, some fruits, and legumes, as well as low-carb fiber sources such as asparagus, broccoli, cauliflower, and berries.

Breakfast may consist of a leafy green vegetables and egg with avocado and berries; lunch could include potato packed with vegetables, beans, and shredded chicken, and supper could consist of a salmon filet or baked tofu with stir-fried broccoli and whole grain rice.

Focus on a single feast if you're not used to cooking or grocery shopping. Shop for supplies for a few breakfast or supper dishes for the week at the grocery shop. Once that becomes a routine, add more feast until you are preparing the majority of your meals at home.

Healthy Eating Suggestions

Here are some practical suggestions to help you start with healthy eating:

- **Make plant-centric foods a priority:** Plant foods such as veggies, fruits, legumes, and almonds should comprise the majority of your diet. Try to include these meals, particularly veggies and fruits, at every feast and snack.

- **Make meals at home:** Cooking at home allows you to broaden your diet. If you're used to getting food delivered or eating out, start by preparing just one or two meals each week.

- **Go grocery shopping regularly:** If you have nutritious goods in your kitchen, you're more prone to prepare healthy meals and snacks. To have healthful products on hand, make one or two supermarket excursions every week.

- **Be aware that your diet will not be ideal:** The crucial word is progress, not perfection. Meet yourself exactly where you stand. Cooking one veggie-packed dinner each week is considerable improvement if you presently dine out every night.

"Cheat days" are not permitted. If your present diet includes "cheat days" or "cheat meals," this indicates an imbalanced diet. There's no need to cheat if you realize that all meals may be part of a healthy diet.

- **Avoid sugar-sweetened beverages:** Limit your consumption of beverages such as soda, energy drinks, and sugary coffees as much as possible. Taking sugary beverages regularly may be harmful to your health.

- **Select filling meals:** When you're hungry, your objective should be to eat full, healthy items rather than consume the fewest carbs possible. Select protein- and fiber-rich meals and snacks that will keep you filled.

- **Consume complete foods:** A healthy diet should consist mostly of natural foods such as vegetables, fruits, legumes, almonds, grains, and proteins such as eggs and fish.

- **Hydrate astutely:** Staying hydrated is a crucial element of good nutrition, and water is the utmost method to do so. If you're not used to drinking water, invest in a sustainable water bottle and savor it with fruit slices or a little lemon.

- **Respect your dislikes**: Don't eat anything if you've tried it multiple times and don't like it. Instead, there are plenty of healthful foods to pick from. Don't push yourself to consume something simply because it's healthy.

These suggestions might help you in making the transition to a healthy diet.

You can also contact with a trained dietitian if you're unsure how to begin adjusting your diet. A dietician can help you in developing a long-term, balanced eating plan that fits your requirements and schedule.

CHAPTER 3

Consuming fruits

Fruit is extremely filling. If you're trying to lose weight, erasing some of your calorie-dense foods for lower-calorie options like fruit may help. During your break, this could mean choosing an orange instead of a granola bar. Consuming fruit may lower the risk of cardiovascular disease.

Consuming a variety of nutritious fruits supplies the body with nutrients and antioxidants that can improve overall health. Oranges, blueberries, apples, avocados, and bananas are all good options, but there are many others.

Fruits are high in fiber and high in important vitamins and minerals. Fruits also contain a range of antioxidants that promote health, such as flavonoids. Eating a fruit and vegetable-rich diet can reduce a person's risk of developing heart issues, cancer, inflammation, and diabetes. Orange and berries may be especially effective in disease prevention.

Nutritious fruits and how to eat them

1. Lemons

Lemons are a citrus fruit with numerous health benefits that are frequently used in traditional remedies. They contain vitamin C and other antioxidants, as do other citrus fruits.

Human health requires antioxidants. These compounds forage free radicals in the body, which can harm cells and lead to diseases like cancer.

Citrus fruits, including lemons, contain phytochemicals, which are active components that benefit health. Among these are:

- Vitamin C
- Folate
- Potassium
- pectin

In grams (g) or milligrams (mg), one 48 g lemon juice contains the following nutrients:

- 10.6 cal

- 3.31 g carbohydrate

- 49.4 milligrams of potassium

- Vitamin C (18.6 mg)

- Calcium: 2.88 mg

- 0.1 g dietary fiber

Lemons are also high in thiamin, riboflavin, niacin, vitamin B-6, folate, and A.

How to consume Them

Use lemon juice to flavor water or squeeze it over a salad or fish.

To calm a sore throat, add a teaspoon of honey to boiling water.

Organic lemon rind can also be consumed.

2. Strawberries

Strawberries are a juicy red fruit that is high in water. Per serving, the seeds contain a lot of dietary fiber. Strawberries are high in antioxidants and vitamins.

They are especially high in anthocyanins, which are flavonoids that can help improve heart health. Strawberries' fiber and potassium content can also help keep your heart healthy. Quercetin is a flavonoid found in strawberries and other colorful berries. This is an anti-inflammatory natural compound.

One cup (150 g) of strawberries provides the following nutrients:

- 48 calories
- 11.5 g dietary fiber
- Calcium 24 mg
- 19.5 milligrams magnesium
- 230 milligrams potassium
- Vitamin C: 88.2 mg

Strawberries are also high in thiamin, riboflavin, niacin, folate, and the vitamins B-6, A, and K.

How to consume strawberry

Strawberries are a fruit that can be used in a variety of ways. They can be eaten raw, mixed into cereal or yogurt, blended into a smoothie, or made into jam.

3. Oranges

Oranges are a nutrient- and mineral-rich citrus fruit with a sweet, round shape.

Oranges are high in vitamin C, with one medium fruit providing 78% of a person's daily value.

A 140 g orange also contains:

- 65 calories
- Carbohydrate 16.5 g
- Fiber (2.8 g)
- Calcium 60.2 mg
- 15 milligrams of magnesium
- 232 milligrams potassium
- Vitamin C 82.7 mg

In the body, vitamin C acts as a powerful antioxidant. This vitamin is also necessary for the immune system to function properly. It strengthens the immune system by assisting the body in absorbing iron from plant-based foods.

Because the human body cannot produce vitamin C, people must obtain it from their diet. Oranges are also high in pectin, a fiber that can help keep the colon healthy by binding to cancer-causing chemicals and removing them from the colon.

Oranges are also high in the following vitamins:

- Vitamin A is a compound necessary for good skin and vision.

- Vitamin B, such as thiamin and folate, aid in the health of the nervous and reproductive systems as well as the production of red blood cells.

How to consume orange

People can eat oranges as a snack or drink a glass of pure orange juice. Make your orange juice or select a brand of fresh juice that is not from concentrate.

To add flavor to a salad, yogurt, or cereal, people can grate orange peel.

4. Limes

Lime is a sour citrus fruit with numerous health benefits.

Lime, like other citrus fruits, is high in vitamin C. They also have antibacterial and antioxidant properties.

One lime juice contains the following nutrients:

- 11 calories
- 3.7 g carb
- 61.6 g calcium
- 3.52 mg of magnesium
- 51.5 milligrams of potassium
- 13.2 milligrams of vitamin C

How to consume Lime

Limes go well with savory dishes. To flavor salad dressings or rice dishes, try incorporating lime juice or grated peel. Alternatively, for a refreshing drink, juice a lime and add it to hot or cold water.

5. Grapefruit

Grapefruits are sour fruits high in vitamins and minerals that promote good health. Grapefruits come in pink, red, or white varieties.

Half a grapefruit (154 g) has the following nutrients:

- 64.7 kilocalories
- 164 g carb
- 2.46 grams fiber
- Calcium 33.9
- Magnesium 13.9

- 208 grams of potassium

Grapefruit flavonoids have been shown to help protect against certain cancers, inflammation, and obesity. Grapefruit furanocoumarins can help protect against oxidative stress and tumors, and they may support bone health.

Grapefruit furanocoumarins may have anticancer properties, particularly in the treatment of breast cancer, skin cancer, and leukemia.

You should consult with your doctor before incorporating grapefruit into your diet because it can interact with certain medications.

How to consume Grapefruit

Try adding grapefruit slices to a fruit salad or squeezing the juice into water for a refreshing drink.

6. Blackberries

Blackberries, like other berries, contain anthocyanins, which are beneficial to one's health.

Because blackberries have a lot of seeds, they have a lot of fiber. This means they can benefit both gut and cardiovascular health.

A half-cup (75 g) serving of blackberries contains the following nutrients:

- 32.2 kilocalories
- 7.21 g dietary fiber
- 3.98 g carbohydrate
- 21.8 milligrams calcium
- Magnesium 15 mg
- 122 milligrams of potassium
- Vitamin C 15.8 mg

How to consume Blackberries

People can eat blackberries fresh, in yogurt for breakfast or dessert, or in smoothies.

7. Apples

Apples are a fast and simple way to add range to your diet. To reap the most health benefits, eat them with the skin on.

Apples are high-fiber fruits, so eating them may help with heart health and weight loss. Apple pectin promotes good gut health.

Apple consumption regularly may reduce the risk of cardiovascular disease, certain cancers, and diabetes.

Apples also contain a high concentration of quercetin, a flavonoid with anti-cancer properties. Individuals who consume whole apples are less likely to be obese than those who do not. Diabetes and heart disease can be diminish as a result of this.

One medium apple, skin on, contains the following nutrients:

94.6 cal

25.1 g of carbs

4.37 g fiber

195 milligrams potassium

10.9 milligrams of calcium

Vitamin C: 8.37 mg

How to consume Apple

Raw apples are an excellent snack, and combining them with almond butter aids to balance protein and fat consumption.

People can also cook with applesauce or add raw or stewed apples to yogurt.

8. Pomegranate

Pomegranates are considered a "superfood" by some because they are high in antioxidants and polyphenols, which aid in the counter against oxidative stress, which can cause disease in the body. Pomegranates have anti-inflammatory properties and may help shield against brain-related illnesses such as Alzheimer's and Parkinson's. This could be due to pomegranates' high polyphenol content.

Human prostate cancer cells may be inhibited in their growth by pomegranates.

One (282 g) raw Pomegranate contains the following nutrients:

- 234 calories
- 52.7g carb
- 11.3g fiber
- Potassium 666mg
- Calcium 28.8mg
- Vitamin C 28.8mg

A pomegranate also has 46.2 micrograms (mcg) of vitamin K in one serving. This vitamin is required for healthy blood cells and strong bones.

How to consume Pomegranate

Pomegranates go well with salads, couscous, and rice dishes.

Because pomegranates are sweet, they can be added to yogurt or fruit salads.

9. Pineapple

Pineapple is an exotic fruit that may aid in inflammation reduction and bowel health. Because of its potential health benefits, pineapple consist an active compound called bromelain, which a lot of people take as a nutritional supplement. Bromelain may be beneficial in the treatment of nasal inflammation or sinusitis.

Manganese, which the body uses to create bone and tissue, is found in pineapples.

A 166-gram slice of pineapple contains the following nutrients:

- 83 cal
- 21.7 g dietary fiber
- Fiber: 2.32 g
- 181 milligrams of potassium
- Vitamin C: 79.3 mg
- Calcium 21.6 mg
- Manganese, 1.54 mg

How to Consume Pineapple

Fresh pineapple can be consumed on its own or in fruit salads. Pineapple can also be used to make tropical salsa or as a topping for fish tacos.

Smoothies can benefit from the addition of frozen pineapple.

10. Bananas

The high potassium content of bananas is well known. One banana (126 g) has approximately 451 mg of potassium. The body uses potassium to regulate blood pressure.

Bananas are also high in energy, with one banana providing 112 calories and 28.8 g of carbohydrates. A banana's 3.28 g of fiber may also aid in regular bowel movements.

A banana contains the following nutrients as well:

- 1.37g protein

- Calcium 6.3mg
- 34 milligrams of magnesium
- 11 milligrams of vitamin C

How to Consume Bananas

A banana can be used to thicken a smoothie. They can also be used as a natural sweetener in baking, such as banana bread or pancakes.

11. Avocado

Avocados are considered a superfood by some due to their health benefits.

Avocados contain a lot of oleic acid, which is a type of monounsaturated fat. Monosaturated fats can aid in cholesterol reduction. Maintaining healthy cholesterol levels through the consumption of healthy lipids can reduce the risk of heart illness and stroke.

Avocados, like bananas, have a high potassium content. They also have lutein, an antioxidant that is beneficial to the eyes and skin.

One avocado (201 g) has the following nutrients:

- 322 calories

- 4.02 g of protein

- 17.1 grams of carbohydrate

- 13.5g dietary fiber

- Calcium: 24.1mg

- Magnesium 58.3mg

- 975 milligrams potassium

- Vitamin C 20.1mg

Avocados are also high in folate, A, and beta-carotene.

How to consume Avocado

Avocado can be added to salads or made into guacamole with Lime, garlic, and tomatoes.

Avocado can be added to smoothies or hummus, or it can be used in baking instead of other fats.

12. Blueberries

Blueberries have numerous health advantages.

Blueberries, like strawberries, contain anthocyanin, which is a potent antioxidant. As a result, they may offer protection against heart disease, stroke, cancer, and other diseases.

Blueberries contain pterostilbene, a compound that may helps in the prevention of deposits buildup in the arteries.

A half-cup (75 g) of blueberries contains the following nutrients:

- 42.8 kcal
- 10.9 g dietary fiber
- 4.5 mg calcium
- 57.8 mg potassium
- 7.28 mg of vitamin C

How to consume Blueberries

Blueberries, whether fresh or frozen, make an excellent addition to breakfast cereals, desserts, yogurt, or smoothies.

The Advantages of Eating Fruit

1. They are an excellent inceptions of vitamins, minerals, and phytonutrients. Eating a fruit salad with a variety of fruits can help boost the body's energy and health.

2. Reducing the risk of cardiovascular disease: Fruits also lower the risk of heart disease and even cancer. Fruits such as apricots, apples, and grapefruit are high in flavonoids, carotenoids, fiber, potassium, and magnesium, all of which protect the heart from a variety of diseases.

3. High in fiber: The presence of dietary fiber in fruits can help to keep blood cholesterol levels in check while also lowering the dangers of adiposity and type 2 diabetes in individuals. Fruits high in fiber, such as strawberries, apples, bananas, and mangos, are also anti-carcinogenic.

4.Fruits contain folate (folic acid), which aids the body in the formation of red blood cells. Pregnant women should consume fruits (orange and grapefruit) in adequate amounts to provide their bodies with folic acid. It assists in lowering the risk of physical and mental deformities in the fetus.

5. Controls blood pressure: Fruits high in potassium, such as bananas, oranges, and avocados, can help you maintain normal blood pressure. They are also low in carbohydrates and fat, making them healthier than any other food substitute.

6. Controls body weight: Fruits high in vitamin C help control body weight. Furthermore, fruits contain no saturated fats or cholesterol, both of which are detrimental to cardiac health.

7. Aids digestion: Fruits high in fiber retain laxative properties and aid digestion in the human body. This also prevents kidney stones from forming.

8.They are high in antioxidants, which help the skin maintain its radiance and glow. Fruits such as papaya, coconut, and others can help with a variety of dermatological conditions. Vitamin A-rich fruits make hair look lustrous.

9. Hydrates the body: Because most fruits are high in water, they are an easy and quick source of hydration. Their intake is critical both in the summer and in the winter.

10. Improves immunity: Fruits are high in calcium, magnesium, and even essential vitamins like vitamin K and vitamin E, which can treat a variety of chronic diseases and boost our resistance to germs and diseases.

CHAPTER 4

The Dangers of Dieting

Diet trends have altered most people's perceptions of weight loss. It's become simple to adhere to various diet plans to meet the demands of society's perception of what is healthy. People, however, frequently fail to recognize the significance of food rules and restrictions. Some diets may work for some people, but they may not work or provide the same benefits for everyone. It's critical to remember that dieting can have unanticipated health consequences.

In most cases, pondering dieting conjures up images of a difficult eating plan to lose weight. Dieting has been repositioned in health and wellness marketing to refer to specific food groups that are low in calories. It can put pressure on you to focus on quick-fix weight loss solutions that come with restrictions and potential control issues.

However, this is one perspective on dieting. A diet, on the other hand, can refer to holistic nutrition. This entails a strategy centered on nourishing your body and mind. As a result, whether you eat healthy or unhealthy foods can have a significant impact on your mental and physical health. Your body requires specific nutrients to function properly. When you don't eat a well-balanced diet, you put yourself at risk for a variety of health problems. Good health and nutrition are important factors in preventing diabetes, cancer, and heart disease.

Experts recommend a well-balanced diet that includes:

Drink plenty of water.

Broccoli and spinach are examples of leafy vegetables.

Eating whole grains can help you get more fiber.

Dairy products are high in calcium.

Poultry products, such as chicken, contain lean protein.

Dieting's Potential Risks
- **Insufficient energy levels**

Carbohydrates are required by your body to provide energy. If you are on a low-carb diet, you may experience a decrease in energy levels. Optimal energy production must consume the recommended amount of healthy carbohydrates, such as whole grains.

- **Digestive problems**

Some fiber-rich foods may be restricted to specific low-carb diets, such as the ketogenic diet. Moving from animal protein and processed foods to plant-based foods, on the other hand, can cause digestive conundrum. Digestive conundrum, such as constipation and diarrhea, can result from digestive issues.

- **Unhealthy food relationship**

You may develop an unhealthy relationship with food if you follow a strict diet with no flexibility in how you eat. In the worst-case scenario, failing to allow for a healthy balance in your diet can lead to an eating disorder. Dieting should be approached with caution because it can lead to an unhealthy infatuation with food and pose potential health risks.

- **A scarcity of nutritious foods**

Some diet plans require you to avoid dairy and grains. A lack of these foods can reduce calcium, protein, and other important minerals and vitamins your body requires. Nutrient deficiency can cause a variety of nutritional deficiencies that affect how your body functions.

- **Hormonal discord**

Any diet that restricts carbohydrate intake can put your hormone production under strain. A low carbohydrate diet can aggravate pre-existing hormone-related conditions such as hyperthyroidism. Furthermore, a low-fat diet can reduce significant hormones and long-term endocrine system issues.

Diet trends can be harmful to one's health because they frequently eliminate essential nutrients. Diet trends may result in the following symptoms:

- Water deficiency.

- Weakness and exhaustion.

- Nausea and migraines.

- Digestion problems.

- Inadequate intake of vitamins and minerals.

Diet trends that severely constrain food groups or nutrients may also mean that you miss out on the health benefits that a well-balanced diet provides.

Diet pressure is something you don't need in your life.

It is not difficult to modify your lifestyle to maintain a healthy weight.

A healthy eating plan will improve your mood and give you more energy.

A well-balanced diet

There is an eating plan that works. You can attain and maintain a healthy body weight without restricting your diet because you can eat everything in moderation. It's known as a balanced eating plan, and it's not a new concept. It will change your life when combined with moderate physical activity.

What you leave out of a balanced eating plan makes all the difference. To be successful with a balanced eating plan, you must:

• Consume an abundance of vegetables, legumes, and fruits.

• Consume a variety of cereals, preferably wholegrain (including loaves of bread, rice, pasta, and noodles).

• Include lean meat, fish, poultry, or substitutes.

• Include milk, yogurt, cheese, or other dairy alternatives.

• Drink lots of water.

• Eat less saturated fat and more total fat.

• Wherever possible, choose low-fat versions of foods.

• Choose low-salt foods.

• If you opt to drink, keep your alcohol intake to a minimum.

• Limit your intake of sugars and sugar-containing foods and beverages. Limit sugar-sweetened beverages in particular.

It can be difficult at first to change your eating and physical activity habits. However, once you've started, it's simple to keep going. Here are some pointers to help with the transition:

• Balance an vigorous lifestyle with a healthy diet.

• Make small, sustainable changes to your lifestyle and eating habits.

• Consume low-calorie, nutritious foods.

• Maintain moderate portion sizes.

• Eat until you are satisfied, not until you are full.

• Make every effort to avoid eating when you are not hungry.

• Recognize that you may be hungrier on some days than others.

• Eat slowly and thoroughly.

• Consume three dishes a daily: breakfast, lunch, and dinner.

• Reduce the amount of 'extra' or 'occasional' foods you consume.

Biscuits, cakes, desserts, pastries, soft drinks, and high-fat snack items such as crisps, samosas, pasties, sausage rolls, other takeaway foods, lollies, and chocolate are examples of 'sometimes' foods.

CHAPTER 5

Increase Your Vegetable Intake

Vegetables are high in dietary fiber, a kind of carbohydrate that helps in the passage of food through the digestive tract. All veggies include beneficial vitamins, minerals, and dietary fiber, but some are particularly beneficial. Eating veggies has health advantages; persons who consume fruits and veggies as part of a whole diet are less likely to have certain diseases. Vegetables give nutrients that are essential for the body's health and upkeep.

Depending on their diets, general health, and nutritional demands, various vegetables may provide a lot of health benefits to particular people.

The Advantages of Eating Vegetables

 All food and beverage options are important. Concentrate on diversity, quantity, and nutrition.

• Eating items with fewer calories per cup, such as vegetables, instead of higher-calorie meals, as part of a balanced diet may help you reduce your calorie consumption.

• consuming a diet heavy in vegetables and fruits as part of a healthy overall diet may lower the risk of heart disease, including heart attack and stroke.

   • It may protect against some forms of cancer.

• Including veggies boosts fiber and potassium levels.

• Eating veggies protects your eyes.

• Aids in skin care by keeping the skin moisturized.

• Vegetables are abundant in fiber and minerals while being low in calories.

• Vegetables are high in cancer-fighting minerals and antioxidants, which may lower your chance of developing some forms of cancer.

• Vegetables help your immune system stay robust.

Vegetables that are good for you:

1. Swiss chard

Swiss chard is another type of leafy green vegetable that is heavy in calcium, vitamins, iron, and antioxidants. Swiss chard is an excellent complement to any vegetarian or vegan diet due to its heavy iron and calcium levels. One cup of fresh swiss chard is largely water and has just seven calories. It also includes:

• A full day's supply of vitamin K for an adult

• High levels of vitamin A

• C vitamin

• Magnesium is a mineral.

• Folic acid

• Iron

• Magnesium

• Antioxidant

Vitamin K is vital for a healthy body, especially for strong bones, because it enhances calcium absorption. Swiss chard also contains a significant quantity of iron for energy and blood health, as well as a high level of magnesium for muscle and nerve function.

Swiss chard leaves are also high in antioxidants, which may help decrease blood pressure and improve heart health.

If you use blood thinners like lawarin (Coumadin), you should exercise caution when increasing your diet of dark leafy greens. For persons using these drugs, doctors recommend keeping a regular vitamin K consumption throughout time.

How to Consume Swiss chard

Raw spinach is popular in salads, sandwiches, and smoothies. Cooked spinach offers several health advantages and is an excellent complement to pasta meals and soups.

2. Kale

Kale is a famous leafy green vegetable that has several health advantages. It has around seven calories per cup of fresh leaves and enough levels of vitamins A, C, and K. People who have high cholesterol may benefit from kale.

Kale juice has been shown to reduce blood pressure, cholesterol, and blood sugar levels. If you use blood thinners like Coumadin, you should exercise caution when increasing your diet of dark leafy greens. While using these drugs, it is recommended to maintain a steady vitamin K consumption.

How to Consume Kale

Baby kale is commonly used in pasta dishes, salads, and sandwiches. Kale chips and drinks are additional options.

3. Broccoli

Broccoli is a superfood that belongs to the same family as cabbage, kale, and Cauliflower. All of them are cruciferous veggies.

Each cup of chopped and boiled Broccoli includes the following nutrients:

• Approximately 31 calories

• The whole daily need for vitamin K

• Vitamin C at double the daily recommended level

These chemicals may protect cells from DNA damage, render cancer-causing substances inactive, and have anti-inflammatory properties. Human research, on the other hand, has been mixed.

How to consume Broccoli

Broccoli is quite adaptable. It may be roasted, steamed, fried, blended into soups, or eaten warm in salads.

4. Peas

Peas are a starchy, sweet vegetable. They have 134 calories per cooked cup and are high in:

• Fiber, with 9 grams (g) each serving

• Protein, with 9 g each serving

• A, C, and K vitamins

• Specific B vitamins

Green peas are high in plant-based protein, which may be especially advantageous to vegetarians and vegans.

Peas and other legumes include fiber, which helps to maintain regular bowel motions and a healthy digestive tract by supporting beneficial bacteria in the stomach. They are also high in saponins, which are plant chemicals that may help prevent oxidative stress and cancer.

How to Consume Peas

It could be useful to keep a bag of frozen peas on hand and gradually add them to the nutritional profiles of pasta meals, risotto, and curries. A pleasant pea and mint soup may also be enjoyed.

5. Sweet potatoes

Sweet potatoes are a type of base vegetable. A medium sweet potato consists 103 calories and 0.17 g of fat when baked in its skin.

Each sweet potato also provides the following nutrients:

• much more vitamin A than an adult's daily need

• 25% of their vitamin C and B6 needs

• 12% of their potassium needs

• beta carotene, which may enhance eye health and aid in cancer prevention.

Diabetes patients may benefit from eating sweet potatoes. This is because they have a low glycemic index and are high in fiber, which may help manage blood sugar.

How to consume Sweet potato

Bake a sweet potato in its peel and serve with a protein source like fish or tofu for a quick supper.

6. Beets

One cup of raw beets includes the following nutrients:

• 58.5 kilocalories

• 442 mg (milligrams) of potassium

• folate (148 micrograms)

Beets and beet juice are excellent for heart health because they contain heart-healthy nitrates. In healthy persons, drinking 500 g of beet juice dramatically reduces blood pressure.

Diabetes patients may benefit from these veggies as well. Beets consist an antioxidant called alpha-lipoic acid, which may be beneficial to persons suffering from diabetic neuropathy.

How to consume Beets

Beets are naturally sweeter when roasted, but they also taste delicious raw in juices, salads, and sandwiches.

7. Carrots

Each cup of chopped carrots has 52 calories and more than four times the daily required amount of vitamin A in the form of beta-carotene for an adult. Vitamin A is essential for good vision, and taking enough of it may help prevent vision loss.

Certain elements found in carrots may potentially be cancer-fighting.

How to consume carrots

Carrots are incredibly adaptable. They are delicious in casseroles and soups, and they have several health advantages when eaten raw, potentially with a dip like hummus.

8. Fermented Vegetables

Fermented veggies include all of the nutrients found in unfermented vegetables, as well as beneficial bacteria. Probiotics are helpful microorganisms found in the body, as well as some foods and supplements.

Probiotics may assist with irritable bowel syndrome symptoms. They may also help to avoid diarrhea caused by illness or antibiotics.

Some good fermentable veggies include:

• cabbage (as in sauerkraut)

• pickled cucumbers

• carrot

• Brussel sprouts

How To Consume Fermented Vegetables

Fermented veggies are consumed in salads, sandwiches, and as a side dish.

9. Tomatoes

Although tomatoes are technically a fruit, they are commonly treated as vegetables and used in savory meals. Each cup of diced raw tomatoes includes the following nutrients:

32 kilocalories

427 milligrams of potassium

24.7 milligrams of vitamin C

Lycopene, a strong antioxidant, is found in tomatoes. Lycopene may help prevent prostate cancer, while tomatoes' beta carotene also helps fight cancer.

Meanwhile, other powerful antioxidants found in tomatoes, such as lutein and zeaxanthin, may be beneficial to eyesight.

People who consume a lot of these compounds in their diet have a 25% lower chance of getting age-related macular degeneration.

How to consume Tomatoes

Tomatoes may be consume raw or cooked, and cooking them releases more lycopene.

10. Garlic

Garlic has long been used in food and healing. Each garlic clove has just four calories and is deficient in vitamins and minerals.

Garlic, on the other hand, is a natural antibiotic. Allium, a garlic component, maybe the source of its health benefits. More studies will be required to confirm this.

How to Consume Garlic

Because heating garlic lowers its health advantages, it is preferable to consume it raw, such as in bruschetta or dips.

11. Onions

Each cup of chopped onions contains:

• 64 kilocalories

• C vitamin

• B6 vitamin

Manganese is a mineral.

Sulfur compounds are found in onions and other allium plants, including garlic. These chemicals may help prevent cancer.

How to Consume Onions

Onions are simple to include in soups, stews, stir-fries, and curries. Eat them raw to receive the most antioxidants — in sandwiches, salads, and dips like guacamole.

12. Alfalfa sprouts

Alfalfa sprouts have just eight calories per cup and a high vitamin K content. These sprouts also include various substances that are beneficial to one's health, including:

• saponins, a kind of bitter chemical with medicinal properties

• flavonoids, a kind of polyphenol with anti-inflammatory and antioxidant properties.

• phytoestrogens, which are plant chemicals that mimic natural estrogens

Alfalfa sprouts have traditionally been used to cure a range of health ailments, including arthritis and renal difficulties.

Alfalfa sprouts include antioxidants, which are substances that may aid in the prevention of illnesses such as cancer and heart disease.

Eating sprouted legumes like these may provide additional advantages—seeds' protein and amino acid content rise after sprouting or germinating.

Germination may also improve the digestibility and dietary fiber content of alfalfa and other seeds.

How to Consume Alfalfa Sprouts

Alfalfa sprouts are contemporary in salads and sandwiches.

13. Bell peppers

Sweet bell peppers come in red, yellow, or orange varieties. Unripe green bell peppers are also popular but have a less sweet flavor.

A cup of diced bell pepper has the following nutrients:

39 kilocalories

Vitamin C (190 mg)

Vitamin B6 (0.434 mg)

folic acid

beta carotene, which is converted by the body into vitamin A

Bell peppers include the following antioxidants and bioactive chemicals:

Dehydroascorbic acid is a kind of vitamin C.

- carotenoid pigments

- C vitamin

- beta carotenoid

- flavonoids, which include quercetin and kaempferol

How to Consume Bell Peppers

Bell peppers are incredibly adaptable and may be easily used for spaghetti, scrambled eggs, or a salad. They're also good sliced with guacamole or hummus on the side.

14. Cauliflower

One cup of chopped Cauliflower has the following nutrients:

- 27 kilocalories

- plenty of vitamin C

- K vitamin

- fiber

Consuming 25 g of dietary fiber every day to improve heart and digestive health. Cauliflower and other cruciferous vegetables also contain the antioxidant indole-3-carbinol. Cauliflower, like Broccoli, includes another component that may help fight cancer: sulforaphane.

How to consume Cauliflower

Raw Cauliflower may be blended to produce cauliflower rice or uscd as a pizza foundation for a low-calorie, warming meal.

Cauliflower may also be eaten in curries or roasted with olive oil and garlic.

15. Seaweed

Seaweed, commonly known as sea vegetables, is an adaptable and nutritious plant with several health advantages. Seaweeds that are commonly seen include:

• kelp

• nori

• sand lettuce

• chlorella

Spirulina is a kind of algae.

• wakame

One of the few vegetable-based sources of omega-3 fatty acids docosahexaenoic acid and eicosatetraenoic acid is seaweed. These are necessary for good health and are largely found in meat and dairy.

Each seaweed has a somewhat distinct nutritional profile, but they are all high in iodine, which is necessary for thyroid function. Eating a variety of sea veggies can offer the body several vital antioxidants that can help minimize cellular damage.

Furthermore, several forms of seaweed include chlorophyll, a plant pigment with anti-inflammatory qualities.

Fucoxanthin is another powerful antioxidant found in brown sea vegetables, such as kelp and wakame. This antioxidant power is 13.5 times that of vitamin E.

How to Consume Seaweed

To prevent introducing too much iodine into the diet, use organic seaweed and eat minimal portions.

Sea veggies are delicious in sushi and miso soups and as a spice for other foods.

CHAPTER 6

Meal planning revitalizes everything.

Choosing what to eat every day may be difficult, especially when you're already balancing your job, family, and social responsibilities. Healthy eating is not something that happens by chance. Instead, we must prioritize nutrition and plan (a little or a lot) to ensure success.

Meal planning is the act of deciding on meals ahead of time. Meal planning is the process of deciding on meals ahead of time based on your schedule, preferences, foods on hand, seasonal produce, sale products, and so on. As a result, meal planning typically leads to weekly grocery shopping for only the things required. You may make your weekly food plans if you know how to meal plan.

Meal Planning Influencing Factors

• Age of family member: Each family member's dietary demands are influenced by his or her age. Children, adolescents, adults, and the elderly are all included.

• Each family member's occupation or activities: A person's employment affects his dietary requirements.

• Family members' health issues: specific meals are not appropriate for specific health conditions.

• Family size: The amount of meals to plan for is determined by the size of the family.

• Season of the year: The majority of foods are seasonal. Food in season is less expensive, fresher, and tastier than food out of season.

• Financial resources

• Availability of time

Meal Planning Recommendations

• The meal must contain all of the required nutrients.

• Include all family members' dietary requirements in the meal plan.

• Change up your diet to avoid boredom.

• Make use of seasonal foods.

• Purchase high-quality meals.

• Plan meals many days in advance to save money and time.

What is the Meal Planning Process?

Meal planning entails the following steps:

• Keeping track of your groceries

• Examining timetables and cooking times

• Meal planning for the week

• Making a grocery list

• Planned grocery shopping and cooking.

3 Professional Meal Planning Tips

1. Make a grocery list.

To begin meal planning, open your refrigerator and conduct a grocery inventory. As a result, you may use your current fresh goods first and just buy what you need at the grocery shop. Furthermore, by using what you have, this first step helps inspire your meals, reduce food waste, and save you money.

Dietitian Tip: Plan your meals BEFORE you go grocery shopping. You may save time and money by purchasing what you require.

2. Examine Schedules and Cooking Time

Meal preparation is constantly giving yourself time to evaluate your calendar ahead of time so you know when you can prepare or batch-cook. For the second meal planning suggestion, I recommend taking 20 to 30 minutes to think calmly about the week ahead, your schedule, and how much time you have to prepare during the week. It is critical to be able to view your timetable. Then, set aside some time each week to plan your meals.

First, make a list of your weekly responsibilities and a realistic estimate of how much time you'll spend cooking that day.

3. Make shopping lists, be creative, and have fun.

Now that your meal plan includes your timetable restrictions for cooking time and your grocery inventory for what you need to use up, it's time to get creative and create those meals! The process of meal planning is more significant than the amount of proficiency in your meals for beginners. In other words, creating a simple meal plan and sticking to it is more essential than attempting complicated culinary inventions. After all, with a hectic nightly schedule, these dinners may be unsustainable. Keeping things simple may be effective.

Dietician Tip: Make a grocery list organized by store categories (for example, vegetables, meat, eggs, seafood, cheese, bakery, grocery (fridge or freezer), and grocery (dry goods). As a result, all produce products are listed together so that you may quickly gather them and go on to the next area. Shopping using a shopping list reduces impulsive purchases and saves money.

The Advantages of Meal Planning

• UNDERSTAND PORTION CONTROL

You'll be able to observe how much you're consuming if you plan your meals. This also prevents you from overeating at restaurants, where the portions are usually much larger than you should be consuming.

• EAT RIGHT

When you're hungry and your blood sugar dips, you're more likely to consume everything you can get your hands on as soon as possible. This is why some of us go to the nearest fast-food restaurant with unhealthy selections. When you have a balanced dinner at your fingertips, full of nutrient-dense food, cooked and ready to go, meal planning solves this issue!

"If we take the time to plan meals, make a grocery list, and keep fruits, veggies, healthy grains, and beans on hand, they will become more handy and consumed more frequently."

• TIME SAVINGS

It's difficult to be hungry and realize you have nothing planned. Instead of staring at your fridge or cupboard, pondering what to make, you can have a nutritious dinner ready in minutes. This also eliminates the need to clean up after cooking.

• MONEY SAVINGS

Everyone can agree that we all attempt to save money, and meal planning is a terrific method to assist. While you avoid spending money at restaurants, meal planning also entails purchasing products in bulk, which can be a significant money saver. Sticking to the list also prevents impulsive purchases at the grocery store.

• AVOID FOOD DISSIPATE

When it comes to meal planning, you go to the grocery shop with a plan and an idea of how you'll use each item. You won't have to worry about food going to waste when every meal has a function.

Whether you're cooking for your full family or just yourself, planning your meals for the week ahead is worthwhile. The trick is to set aside a small amount of time each week to accomplish it.

CONCLUSION

In conclusion, healthy eating habits are crucial in sustaining good health and preventing chronic diseases. Developing healthy eating habits necessitates gradual modifications to your diet and lifestyle. You can build healthy eating habits that improve general well-being by planning meals, cooking at home, consuming more fruits and vegetables, choosing whole grains, and practicing mindful eating.